D1474626

Eat
—— Your ——
Cholesterol

How to Live Off the Fat of the Land and Feel Great!

EAT MEAT, DRINK MILK, SPREAD THE BUTTER -- AND LIVE LONGER...

By **William Campbell Douglass II,** MD

This publication is designed to provide accurate and authoritative information in regard to the subject matter covered. It is sold with the understanding that the publisher is not engaged in rendering medical, or other professional service. If medical advice or other expert assistance is required, the services of a competent professional person should be sought. This book is not a substitute for medical advice.

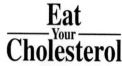

Eat
—Your—
Cholesterol
How to Live Off the Fat of the Land
and Feel Great!

**EAT MEAT, DRINK MILK, SPREAD THE BUTTER
-- AND LIVE LONGER...**

Copyright © 1994, 2003
by
William Campbell Douglass II, MD

ISBN 9962-636-19-1

Cover illustration by
Alex Manyoma (alex@3dcity.com)

Please, visit Rhino's website for other publications from
Dr. William Campbell Douglass
www.rhinopublish.com

Dr. Douglass' "Real Health" alternative medical newsletter
is available at www.realhealthnews.com

RHINO PUBLISHING, S.A.
World Trade Center
Panama, Republic of Panama

Voicemail/Fax
International: + 416-352-5126
North America: 888-317-6767
P.O. Box 025724
Attention PTY 5048
Miami, Fl. 33102 USA

Contents

Introduction 1

Chapter 1
The Battle Is On 5
    This Means War... 6
    The Propaganda Blitz 7
    They've Even Fooled the *Journal*.................. 9

Chapter 2
The Facts About Cholesterol 15
    The Great Butter Battle................................ 19
    More Evidence... 21
    The Battle Continues 23
    Everything's Better with Butter on It 24
    Don't Stare.. 26
    More About Veggie Oil 32
    Scammery.. 36

Chapter 3
Count Your Eggs....................................... 39
    "Where's the Beef?" 43
    Commonly Consumed Protein 49
    The Chicken Scoop 50

Chapter 4
A Bit of History 51
    Monkey Business 52
    Living off the Fat of the Land in Africa 54
    Action to Take... 59

Suggested Further Reading 63

Other Books by
William Campbell Douglass, MD

- *Add 10 Years To Your Life*

- *Aids And Biological Warfare*

- *Bad Medicine*

- *Color Me Healthy*

- *Dangerous Legal Drugs: The Poisons In Your Medicine Chest*

- *Dr. Douglass Complete Guide To Better Vision*

- *The Milk Book -- How Science Is Destroying Nature's Nearly Perfect Food*

- *Grandma Bell's A To Z Guide To Healing*

- *Hormone Replacement Therapies: Astonishing Results For Men And Women.*

- *Hydrogen Peroxide - Medical Miracle*

- *Into The Light - Tomorrow's Medicine Today*

- *Lethal Injections - Why Immunizations Don't Work*

- *Painful Dilemma -- Patients In Pain -- People In Prison*

- *Prostate Problems: Safe, Simple Effective Relief*

- *St. Petersburg Nights*

- *Stop Aging Or Slow The Process: Exercise With Oxygen Therapy*

- *The Eagle's Feather*

- *The Joy Of Mature Sex And How To Be A Better Lover...*

- *The Smoker's Paradox: The Health Benefits Of Tobacco*

Introduction

How to Live Off
the Fat of the Land
and Feel Great!

A young American was taking a course in a French cooking school and, after a meat-cooking demonstration, asked the chef-teacher: "What about all that cholesterol and fat?" The chef replied with his nose tilted upward, "Monsieur, I am a chef, not a physician." Strange as it may seem, this chef is probably a better physician than those in the American Medical Association, at least where cholesterol is concerned. Why? Because when it comes to high-cholesterol cooking, the French ignore the American fat phobia and go hog wild.

One of France's leading chefs said it best: "Without butter and cream, why come to France?"

You can do without some wonderful fat-laden food if you want to, but it's not going to prolong your life, and you'll miss some fantastic meals.

It was the French who invented Bearnaise sauce -- three egg yolks and a half pound of butter -- and then seized upon the idea of pouring it over a nice fat-marbled filet mignon. With the steak they eat a flaky croissant, slathered with fresh, creamy butter. In southern France they eat duck fat *instead* of butter. And they consume enormous quantities of cheese that has a higher cholesterol and saturated fat content than beef or pork. (Charles de Gaulle once said, "How can you be expected to govern a country that has 246 kinds of cheese?")

In fact, the typical French diet would strike terror into the heart of any doctor in the United States. But here's the bottom line: *The French* have the lowest rate of heart disease of any western industrialized nation -- so pass the *saucisses de Toulouse.* No, on second thought, make it the *boudins maison.*

In spite of such facts, Americans are being saturated with anti-cholesterol propaganda. If you watch very much television, you're probably one of the millions of Americans who now has a terminal case of cholesterol phobia. The propaganda is relentless and is often designed to produce fear and loathing of this worst of all food contaminants. You never hear the food propagandists bragging about their product being fluoride-free or aluminum-free, two of our truly serious food-additive problems. But cholesterol, an essential nutrient, not proven to be harmful in any quantity, is constantly pilloried as a menace to your health. If you don't use corn oil, Fleischmann's margarine, and Egg Beaters, you're going straight to atherosclerosis hell with stroke, heart attack, and premature aging -- and so are your kids.

Chapter 1

The Battle Is On

In October 1988, I received a letter from the American Medical Association (AMA) in regard to the new attack on cholesterol. It read: "Dear Dr. Douglass, (I was deeply moved at being remembered after telling them where to put their organization 20 years ago.) In an unprecedented initiative aimed at reducing the incidence of cholesterol-linked (heart disease), the AMA has declared war on cholesterol.... We are launching a major multi-faceted, multimedia cholesterol-lowering offensive."

As a result, the bayonets have been fixed, the guns loaded, the propaganda apparatus has been working around the clock, and the troops are eagerly awaiting an all-out attack. This is a war on the insidious and pernicious enemy: Cholesterol! It's a 5-pronged attack

(How can it fail?) led by the AMA, the pharmaceutical industry, the federal government, the food industry, and the press. They are determined to spoil all of your fun at the dinner table -- and make you pay dearly for it.

Read the last half of that last sentence again, because the three-letter word "pay" is what this whole war is all about. The more the drug companies, doctors, and anyone else involved in the "war" can blow this out of proportion, the more money they can make. If you don't believe me, let's take a look at the strategy behind the war and then the facts about cholesterol. Then we can all make a better decision about our eating habits.

This Means War

The numbers game is the biggest weapon used by the anti-cholesterol centurions to frighten the populace into a diet fit only for a zebra. These commanders have decreed that the magic number is 200 (mg per deciliter) for blood cholesterol, and the lower the reading the better. But recent exhaustive studies have shown that 250 is a level not associated with any increase in cardiovascular disease. Furthermore, the "lower-the-better", rule is not only bad science, but very dangerous advice. Extremely low cholesterol readings, those in the lower 10 percent of the population, have an increased mortality from all causes. "From all causes" means that, for reasons unknown, those with a very low blood cholesterol level die sooner from accidents, cancer, strokes, lung or kidney disease, etc.

Millions of healthy Americans, frustrated, depressed, and seized with cholesterol phobia, are valiantly trying to beat down their blood cholesterol levels by eating oat bran, grass foods, and anything else that sprouts from Mother Earth. They avoid all the good stuff: eggs, butter, milk, red meat (especially dangerous, we're told), or anything else that bleeds except fish (but don't touch shellfish). As the actors tell you on television commercials, or at least imply, the way to eternal life is through hypocholesterolemia (low cholesterol). Even your doctor believes it.

But how does your doctor explain the huge subset of Americans, 25,000,000 in all, who have a blood cholesterol range from 200 all the way up to 300, and yet are completely free of atherosclerotic heart disease? The group is known as premenopausal women. These "hypercholesterolemic" women are not protected by female hormones, as previously thought. It has to do with iron metabolism, but that's another story. Suffice it to say that iron is likely to be the major factor in atherosclerosis, and cholesterol levels are not a factor at all.

The Propaganda Blitz

As Merck, Sharp & Dohme's (MSD) marketing chief, Jerry Jackson said, "We've had to develop a market as well as develop a drug." And that's exactly what they've done. MSD has produced, under the auspices of the AMA, a very expensive and toxic anti-cholesterol drug called Mevacor. The National Heart, Lung, and Blood Institute (NHLBI) has recommended that doctors go easy on prescribing this powerful drug because, although it's "a major advance," its effects on coronary heart disease incidence and "long-term safety haven't yet been established." (If its safety and effectiveness haven't been established, then how can it be considered a major advance? Is the NHLBI trying to avoid offending a rich and powerful drug company?)

Meanwhile, Merck, Sharp & Dohme has been conducting a brazen TV propaganda blitz to panic the American people into thinking that their blood cholesterol is a sure-fire indicator of their health status and, if the cholesterol is high, certain death is soon to follow. At the end of one of their anti-cholesterol propaganda pieces, the jagged line of a heart monitor goes flat and an alarm whines, indicating that the heart has stopped -- a fatal heart attack. The announcer then intones: "Get your number down before your number's up."

Haven't things gotten out of hand when a drug company can panic people into a doctor's office to demand a dangerous drug for a condition not proven to be alleviated by that drug? A high blood cholesterol level is a *sign* of *disease*, not a disease. Bodily dysfunctions are not cured by treating signs or symptoms. Your doctor wouldn't think, for instance, of treating your bacterial pneumonia with just aspirin. He would be treating just a sign of the disease, fever, and not the infection itself. Does it make any more sense to treat an elevated cholesterol level when we don't know why it is elevated? *It is very possible that the elevated cholesterol is a protective mechanism of the body, and lowering it is the wrong thing to do.*

They've Even Fooled the *Journal*

The propaganda blitz has been so awesome that even the *New England Journal of Medicine (NEJM)*, one of our more scientifically responsible journals, has abandoned science and swallowed the killer-cholesterol line. "The optimal intake of cholesterol," they editorialize, "is probably zero, meaning the avoidance of animal products."

After making this wrong-headed and unscientific statement, they temporize by admitting that "sound data are needed," "The lack of more direct human evidence remains frustrating," "In the absence of fully satisfactory data, ... a reasonable policy would seem to admit uncertainty, ... and we must 'hedge our bets.'" There is a certain wistfulness to this editorial as if they were saying, "Would someone please prove that our dietary recommendations have some scientific justification?"

After all this sophisticated (and sophistic) hand-wringing, the editors admit that "the only dietary factor consistently associated with the risk of coronary heart disease in epidemiologic studies is alcohol...." And that has a powerful *protective effect*.

The editors fatten up their editorial with a swipe at obese people, definitely a persecuted majority. "Obesity is primarily an exercise deficiency syndrome." If so, then why are lazy people, like me, still thin?

The Samburu of East Africa don't read the *New England Journal of Medicine* so they don't know that all the animal fat they eat is bad for them. They will probably outlive the editors of the *NEJM* and, besides, I'd like to see one of those Harvard professors kill a lion with a spear.

There's something in this for everybody, including the doctors. Doctors' waiting rooms often sport fancy wall charts proclaiming the cholesterol bogeyman and there are plenty of free brochures describing the terrible consequences of an elevated cholesterol. All supplied by the friendly snake oil salesmen from Merck, Upjohn, Bristol-Myers, or any of a few dozen other companies on the take for a piece of the burgeoning cholesterol market.

In spite of claims that they are "educating" the public, the drug companies are simply pushing drugs so that panicked patients will pressure their doctor to prescribe this latest life-saving wonder. Many doctors don't have the courage to resist this outrageous interference in the practice of medicine. Besides, it takes time and patience to explain to the patient why a particular drug is not indicated in his case. Some will go along out of fear of losing the patient and, besides, "If I don't give it to them another doctor will."

Dr. Norman Kaplan, a professor at Southwestern Medical School, sums it up: "Aggressive drug-company promotions produce an excessive reliance by doctors on medication when diet and exercise can often be as good. There already is widespread overuse of diabetes and hypertension drugs. I suspect the same thing will happen with cholesterol."

To add to the utter senselessness of the whole anti-cholesterol movement, we now know that the original research by Dr. Anitchkow was irrelevant. He fed cholesterol to rabbits and reported that they developed atherosclerosis. It turns out that if the cholesterol is pure and fresh, it has no effect whatsoever on the arteries of rabbits. In humans, the measurement of blood cholesterol levels is meaningless unless diet and activity are carefully controlled -- and this, in most cases, is impossible.

Perhaps the slickest operators in this cholesterol craze are the boys at Warner-Lambert. Warner-Lambert bombarded doctors with letters telling them that its anti-cholesterol drug, Lopid, "appeared" to reduce second heart attacks. The FDA said that "all claims from the study are premature and unsubstantiated." But that didn't stop Warner-Lambert. With a favorable report published in the trusted *NEJM*, Warner-Lambert started brainwashing the doctors through a prestigious-sounding organization called the International Lipid Information Bureau (ILIB). A spokesperson for ILIB informs us that the bureau is "a clearinghouse for researchers, doctors, and the public." But it is actually nothing but a publicity front created, financed, and directed by Warner-Lambert. Of course, your doctor, busy trying to keep up with the flood of information/propaganda coming into his office, doesn't know that the ILIB is a self-serving marketing tool of Warner-Lambert.

Warner-Lambert brought four Finnish investigators to a giant New York news conference that was so effectively promoted it generated front-page news all over the U.S. Then Warner-Lambert flew the scientists, accompanied by the company's chairman, in its private jet, to a big cardiology meeting in Anaheim, California. Warner-Lambert chairman Joseph Williams honored the researchers at a dinner and gave each of them a souvenir clock from Tiffany (nice!).

In a landmark report in late 1987, the government, through the NHLBI, practically ordered doctors to treat cholesterol levels that had previously been considered normal (anything above 200). This started the drug company stampede that has the American people cholesterol nuts. The American Heart Association, not wanting to appear to be lagging behind the "education" efforts of the pharmaceutical giants, started a program to teach 40,000 doctors how to treat the great cholesterol scourge. What the American Heart Association coyly downplays is that the program is financed by the pharmaceutical giant, Merck, to the tune of $400,000.

I've got more on the Merck propaganda juggernaut, but I'm getting an elevated cholesterol just writing about it. Just to give you an idea of the enormity of this scam, if doctors follow the NHLBI guidelines, 25 percent of American adults will be put on cholesterol-lowering drugs! They will be required to visit their doctor monthly, because the drugs have dangerous side effects, and this will require expensive laboratory testing.

A good example of the astronomical amounts of money involved in this scam is what would happen to the budget of just one average hospital. Dr. Alan K. Halperin, director of the hypertensive clinic at the Veterans Administration Medical Center in Albuquerque, New Mexico, said that if therapy were to be instituted according to the recommended guidelines, the cost would be "absolutely incredible." At the Albuquerque VA hospital, drug treatment conceivably might be indicated for 10,500 patients. At an estimated average annual wholesale drug cost of $400 per patient, this would come to $4.2 million - almost the entire annual pharmacy budget for the hospital. And that is just one of thousands of hospitals. "We are going to break the bank if we follow the guidelines," Halperin added.

Let's look at an even more mind-boggling figure. The cost of extending the life of a 65-year-old man for one year by using cholesterol-lowering drugs (assuming they work) would be $777,600 (and that is not a misprint .

Chapter 2

The Facts About Cholesterol

The truth about cholesterol as it pertains to good health is actually the opposite of what the medical establishment has been saying. Not only have they been selling bad drugs, the anti-cholesterol syndicate has been passing out bad nutritional advice. For instance, did you know that where blood cholesterol is concerned, *most of us are self-regulators?* For most people, telling them to lower their cholesterol intake, even if their cholesterol is elevated, is not justified or scientifically supportable.

Dr. Donald McNamara did a study at Rockefeller University which illustrated the futility of dietary cholesterol restriction. A high cholesterol diet was fed to 50 subjects and most of them responded by absorbing less cholesterol from the intestine. Eight subjects actually showed a decrease in plasma cholesterol on the high cholesterol diet.

Dr. McNamara also observed that the "worst case" diet (a big steak with a half inch of fat around it covered by three eggs -- a real Australian breakfast that has high saturated fat and high cholesterol) compared with a "best case" diet (horse food, rabbit food, egg white, veggies, corn oil, high polyunsaturated fat, and low cholesterol) will result in a cholesterol difference of eight percent. Laboratory error and variation from day to day can be 20 percent or even higher. Now aren't you glad the food companies, the American Medical Association, and the government have issued a billion-dollar propaganda blitz on cholesterol? This cholesterol "war" will result in millions of people, as high as 25 percent of the population, being treated for something they don't have (hyper-cholesterolemia) by a method that is not proven (anti-cholesterol chemotherapy).

Exercise, cold weather, emotion, and type A blood are all related to higher than "normal" blood cholesterol levels. With all of these variables how can they judge the effect of this anti-cholesterol chemotherapy? With only one in 25 people with heart attacks demonstrating an elevated blood cholesterol, what on earth are they going to prove with this unscientific and dangerous experiment? (Doctor to patient: "The bad news is you've had a heart attack and may die. The good news is your cholesterol is normal.")

Dr. John Story, professor of nutrition at Purdue University, backs Dr. McNamara: "Dietary cholesterol isn't a major factor as far as changes in serum cholesterol are concerned." And Dr. McNamara concluded: "We're not going to cure the world of heart diseases by lowering cholesterol levels."

Dr. Earl P. Bendett, of the University of Washington, demonstrated, through the use of electron microscopy, that there is very little cholesterol in the nasty little deposits that clog arteries. Arterial plaques are composed of smooth muscle cells that have migrated from the middle layer (media) of the artery to the inner layer (intima). There were also fibrils and platelets, but very little cholesterol. The next time you are chewing the fat with your doctor, ask him (if you have the nerve) why he is pushing a low-cholesterol diet and drugs that force the cholesterol level down if the clogged arteries don't contain any cholesterol.

Bendett says that the deposits are actually a form of non-invasive cancer and the well-respected medical journal, the *Lancet*, editorialized that a virus may account for Bendett's discovery.

Back to your doctor. When you ask him, "What do you think about the tumorigenic etiology of atherosclerosis?" He will probably reply: "What medical school did you go to?" To which you should reply, "Oh, I've been reading the Lancet since the third grade."

If eating butter caused heart disease, then everyone in Udaipur, India, would have been long dead. They have the highest butter consumption in the world and eat practically nothing but meat and animal fat. Yet, death from heart disease is about the same as it was for Americans at the turn of the century, meaning close to zero. Like the people of Udaipur, Americans ate butter, lard, and more lard in the early 20th century. Since then, margarine and vegetable oil consumption has risen 300 percent -- and heart attacks have gone up 3,500 percent. So what your doctor is innocently and sincerely recommending is probably increasing not only heart disease and cancer (The poly-unsaturated oils are immunosuppressant), but osteoporosis as well.

A tragic illustration of what a strict vegetarian, no-cholesterol diet may do to you is the case of famous basketball star, Bill Walton. Walton was a fanatic about what he considered to be good nutrition. No animal food -- dairy or otherwise - passed his lips. He developed severe osteoporosis and consequent foot and ankle fractures from the constant jumping on hard wood floors required of his sport. A brilliant sports career was finished. Walton, learning from his mistake, became a spokesman for the meat industry.

If your doctor suggests that you lower your cholesterol intake or take Mevacor, Questran, Colestid, Lopid, or some other cholesterol-lowering drug, ask him:

(1) What is his cholesterol level?

(2) Would he take the drug if his cholesterol was at the same level as yours?

(3) Does he really think the drug will improve your health or prolong your life?

(4) Does he own any stock in the company that sells the drug he wants you to take?

(5) Does he do clinical research for that company?

(6) If your doctor's answer to questions (4) and (5) is "yes," then get a second opinion.

The Great Butter Battle

Margarine won the battle for the grocer's shelf long before cholesterol was identified as Public Enemy Number One. If you check your supermarket, you'll see that there is very little space allocated for butter. Pretty soon they'll sell it under the counter and put it in a plain brown wrapper -you wouldn't want your neighbors to know that you are poisoning your family. And trying to find some good pig lard is even harder. In fact, show up with lard or butter and you will probably get a lecture from the checkout girl on "the dangers of saturated fats." Everybody's an expert. And just try to order four eggs for breakfast at Shoney's. They'll probably call the police -- suicide attempt.

It may surprise you to learn that the battle of butter vs. margarine started *over a hundred years ago* in

1886. It was the first great impassioned controversy in the Congress involving a pure food issue. The contest centered around whether margarine should have "equal protection" under tax law with butter. Never before in the history of Congress had there been such an acrimonious and emotional debate over food.

In the original skirmishes, the butter boys won hands down. Senator "Fighting Bob" LaFollette, never at a loss for words, came to the defense of the butter industry: "Ingenuity, striking hands with cunning trickery, compounds a substance to counterfeit an article of food. It is made to look like something it is not; to taste and smell like something it is not; to sell like something it is not; and so deceive the purchaser."

The Great Butter Battle continued into the early 20th century when one North Carolina representative said this "cheap, nasty grease" could be fatal. He warned that many of those who ate margarine might have a coroner's verdict of "died of bogus butter."

With remarkable prescience, which is only now becoming appreciated, D.E. Salmon, chief of the U.S. Bureau of Animal Industry, said that an invention like margarine "which introduces a radical change to the manufacture of an article of food which goes on the table of every family in the land *might produce an unexpected and remarkable effect on the public health.*" (Emphasis added.) These prophetic words were written over 50 years ago.

Others joined the argument and said that "this greasy substitute" had only one advantage over butter and that was price. That was certainly true, but price won out in the long run and, in 1950, after a 64-year battle, the tax was removed from oleo.

People just didn't realize that butter was worth the price because of its superior nutritional quality. Butyric acid, or butyrate, is an edible fatty acid present at the level of four percent in butter. Butyrate is a preferred food by normal cells, so much so that its half life in blood is only five minutes. Butyrate has the wonderful quality of being detrimental to the abnormal physiology of cancer cells. It can be used in the treatment of cancer, but requires a great deal more than that obtained from eating butter: consumed eight to ten grams, four times a day, by mouth or as a two percent buffered intravenous solution. By intravenous, 40 grams per day is the recommended dose. (If I tried to treat you with this method, we'd probably *both* go to jail.)

More Evidence

The nutritional superiority of butter over margarine has been proven beyond a doubt, and with absolutely no evidence that it will raise your cholesterol. One of the earliest and most convincing studies which should have been seen as a warning light by nutritionists, but was ignored, was performed by Dr. T.W. Gullickson, Professor of Dairy Chemistry at the University of Minnesota. The study proved the nutritional superiority of butterfat over vegetable oils, which are the main ingredients of the margarines.

Gullickson was trying to find a cheaper way to raise calves for veal production. He removed the expensive cream from the top of the milk -- for those of you under 40 years of age, milk comes with a cream layer on the top until the farmer smashes it with a homogenizer -- and substituted cheap vegetable oils (tallow, coconut oil, corn oil, cotton seed oil, or soybean oil) to simulate milk. Enough vegetable oil was used in the skimmed milk to imitate the 3.5 percent butterfat of natural milk. If calves would grow on this cheap substitute, the cost of veal could be drastically reduced.

Guess what? Almost all of the calves sickened and died. As often happens in research, Gullickson proved something entirely different from his original objective. He found that calves will only grow on God's own natural milk straight from their mommy, or somebody else's mommy. On Gullickson's corn oil (corn oil is a highly promoted form of margarine), eight out of ten of the calves died in less than six months; some expired just one month after the switch was made.

If vegetable oil products are so devastating to the health of calves, do you suppose they might be bad for humans -- especially children? But even most people living on farms today eat the solidified vegetable oil known as margarine, even though there's a cow right outside the window.

The Battle Continues

As you can see, the downfall of animal fat came about, not as the result of good science, but from effective propaganda. Since 1950, the margarine folks have been winning the battle, but the tide seems to be shifting very slowly. The Associated Press reported on May 16, 1994, "A startling new report out of Harvard University says a little-known type of fat that lurks in margarine and other processed foods could be responsible for 30,000 of the nation's annual heart disease deaths."

In 1993, researchers reported that margarine and "other processed foods" (including baby formula made from highly saturated oils) could double the risk of heart attacks. Dr. Walter Willett, Harvard's chief of nutrition, said the American people are "being grossly misled" on the subject of saturated vegetable oils. Well, I guess better late than never, but Walter, where have you been for the last ten years? Didn't you read my book reporting all of this? I guess not.

Well, the fat's in the fire on this one. I don't know how something can be "startling" when it's been known for well over a hundred years. It's only startling if you have refused to believe what's right before your eyes.

How is the AMA going to extricate itself from this embarrassing mess? After sending out the letter to its members declaring war on cholesterol, the AMA has now found that one of its favorite weapons in this war, margarine, is "worse than butter," as the press puts it. (Butter isn't "worse" than anything. It's a very nutritious food and vital for a balanced diet.)

In response, I'm sure the AMA and the food industry will simply come up with a "new and improved" version of margarine. "We have been killing you with our greasy substitute for butter, but we're not going to do that any more." That's not exactly the way they will promote it. It will be more like: "heart-saver," "less free radicals," *"More HDL," "Less LDL,"* etc., etc.

Everything's Better with Butter on It

The American people (and their doctors) have been sold on the idea that "polyunsaturated" vegetable oils are the key to good health. If this were true, then everybody would be healthy because a more-than-adequate supply of such oils is found in vegetables, nuts, and meat. It would be difficult, even with the lousy average American diet, not to get adequate amounts of unsaturated fats. Man has been eating meat, fat, and dairy products for thousands of years, but hardening of the arteries is a new disease. My father practiced medicine in Georgia 70 years ago and he rarely saw heart attacks. Coronary heart disease has only become common since the advent of margarine and the massive consumption of vegetable oils.

The dramatic increase in heart disease in this century has not been accompanied by an increase in animal fat consumption. But there has been a dramatic increase in the consumption of vegetable fats. The traditional fats, dairy and lard (my Grandma Bell ate lots of lard), have been replaced by Mazola, Puritan, and the other vegetable oils. These oils are "hydrogenated" into a solid state called margarine. This hydrogen bombardment turns the liquid oil into an unnatural product that nature did not intend and, in experimental animals at least, causes cancer and arteriosclerosis.

Corn oil, heavily promoted to reduce cholesterol, actually causes the body to produce more cholesterol than lard. A University of Georgia study in 1972 by Dr. W.O. Caster proved that the more meat fatty acid (stearate) one eats the lower the blood cholesterol. He found that meat fat also lowers the blood pressure. This is exactly the opposite of what you have been told -- we are being killed by a combination of Hollywood hype, Madison Avenue buncombe, junk food medicine men from Nabisco and Harvard, and a bunch of doctors who believe anything the American Heart Association tells them.

Linseed oil and olive oil are exceptions to the above findings. They are not cancer-promoting. Olive oil may even prevent atherosclerosis. Cretan (not cretin) men consume large quantities of olive oil. Fat constitutes 43 percent of the diet in Crete, outrageous according to American experts. Their blood fats and cholesterol remain normal and they have a very high prevalence of centenarians.

It should be noted that the polyunsaturated fats are not directly cancer-causing. They seem to act as co-factors or promoters. So if you are infected with a cancer virus, and millions of people are, excess polyunsaturated vegetable oil in your diet may trigger cancer.

Don't Stare

One of the most convincing studies in this regard was the Irish Brothers Study which was conducted by Fred Stare of Harvard. Thirty years ago, when the study was conducted, the Irish population had a much higher concentration of butter, lard, and other saturated fats, and essentially no margarine or other vegetable fats and oils in their diet as compared to their siblings in Boston, Massachusetts. It was thus assumed that the incidence of cardiovascular disease would be much higher in animal-fat Ireland than in vegetable-fat, cholesterol-free Boston. The findings were exactly opposite. The Irish, living on good old pig fat, and without the benefit of nutritional advice from the dieticians of the American Heart Association, clearly had fewer heart attacks than their brothers in Boston.

Cramming this anti-cholesterol propaganda down the throats of the American people is not just cheap hucksterism and quackery that does most of its harm to the pocketbook. There is strong scientific evidence that increasing the polyunsaturated oils in your diet may make you look older, increase the likelihood of your developing cancer, and cause cardiovascular disease. Margarine, for instance, is subtly and constantly promoted on television and even in doctor's scientific publications as a drug to prevent heart disease. They don't actually come out and say: "Eat this margarine, not evil cholesterol-elevating butter, in order to avoid a heart attack." But the propaganda has worked so effectively that even the doctors have fallen for it. What does the cardiologist (who probably knows less about nutrition than his secretary) tell the patient after a heart attack? Eat margarine, stay away from "red meat" and eat only three eggs a week. Pish posh.

Professor Stare advises people to drink a cup of corn oil once a week for good health. In light of the scientific evidence, this is preposterous nonsense and errant quackery. Doesn't Stare read his own stuff? According to research done at the University of Minnesota, eating large amounts of corn oil will increase the amount of cholesterol in your heart and liver. No wonder Dr. George Mann, one of the truly honest and intelligent clinical nutritionists of our age, said that Stare was a public relations man, not a scientist. In case you're interested, Stare is also a plagiarist and he filched funds from the government that he was forced to pay back. He should have gone to jail.

If you find these revelations on Harvard Professor Fred Stare to be unusual, you shouldn't. His behavior is typical of present-day biomedical science. A bitter Dr. Mann, the distinguished physician and researcher who exposed old Faker Fred, said: "Biomedicine has become an obscene place and I for one am glad that I am about to leave it. A challenging, intellectual, and humanitarian profession has been turned into a crass commercial enterprise.... To support the diet/heart hypothesis, with all its easy money would be a deceit. Saturated fat and cholesterol in the diet are not the cause of coronary heart disease. That myth is the greatest scientific deception of this century, perhaps of any century."

We cannot leave Dr. Mann without a few more paragraphs. His work was pivotal in the diet/heart controversy. He demonstrated 15 years ago that the cholesterol hypothesis was nothing but commercial rubbish and was, in fact, probably dangerous to our health. Dr. Mann discovered a factor in fresh whole milk (which your benevolent government has outlawed) that inhibits the synthesis of cholesterol.

He proved the effect of calories on serum cholesterol levels. Weight gain drives the blood cholesterol up and weight loss will drive it down. This, he says, explains "illusory treatments" such as the Pritikin horse feed diet. Who wouldn't lose weight on such puny rations? It should also be noted that the weight loss brings down the blood cholesterol, but the diet gets the credit. (Pritikin had leukemia and, unlike most grass guzzlers who will eat a steak if someone else is paying for it, must have followed his own bad advice.)

Mann dared to tell the truth. He had the temerity to point out that the cholesterol emperors weren't wearing any clothes. For this honesty he had to pay a price. He was denied research funding by the National Institutes of Health, the American Heart Association, and the other commissars of the medical establishment.

Fred Stare and his ilk at Harvard and other centers of indoctrination are largely responsible for the fact that the American people have tripled their consumption of vegetable oils with a resulting skyrocketing of the incidence of heart disease and other forms of arteriosclerosis.

Consider this seldom-discussed fact: Elevated blood cholesterol levels are most often found *after* a person develops heart disease. So is it not just as likely that the elevated cholesterol is a protective mechanism by the body, attempting to prevent further damage, and that artificially lowering the cholesterol with drugs and a rabbit diet may be exactly the wrong thing to do?

The whole concept of cholesterol depositing on arterial walls and then penetrating through that wall is contrary to biological science as we understand it. Yet, that is the concept most people have about how arteries become clogged. Don't feel bad about it -your doctor thinks the same thing. This cholesterol deposition concept has never been demonstrated and knowledgeable biologists don't even consider it to be a possibility!

Dr. Paul Dudley White is one of the icons of American medicine and was the leading cardiologist of his day. He and Fred Stare practiced on the same hallowed ground of Northeastern academia, but Dr. White was a great clinician and was intellectually honest: "I think I have a pretty clear idea of the role of proteins, carbohydrates, and so forth, but I must admit I'm thoroughly confused about cholesterol and, for that matter, I'm not sure whether some form of the weight-control diets might not be dangerous to the heart. The amount in the blood, we call it serum cholesterol, is not necessarily related to cholesterol found in food."

Dr. White admitted that he was confused. But what about the dieticians who tell you, with the greatest of confidence and backed by the authority of the American Heart Association, not to drink milk, but eat more fish when the fish contains eight times more cholesterol than milk?

You'd almost think that the American Heart Association was out to kill us. They suppress their own funded reports when those studies show the dangers of excessive intake of vegetable oils, they constantly warn of the dangers of traditional foods, especially "red meat" and butter, and they recommend a diet high in vegetable oils that no known human population eats now or has ever eaten. Does that make sense to you? If you follow the advice of the "experts" at the American Heart Association, you will be eating a whopping 15 percent of polyunsaturated fat in your diet. This is guaranteed to make you wizened, cancerous, arteriosclerotic, impotent, and bad-tempered -- and if you eat that way you deserve it.

Am I being extreme in saying the American Heart Association is out to do us in? Dr Denham Harmon of the University of Nebraska School of Medicine, reports that these extreme recommendations for vegetable oil consumption can shorten your life span by 15 years. He found that the more vegetable oil you feed experimental animals the sooner they die. Are you being used by the American Heart Association as an experimental animal?

The NHLBI would have you believe that of the 550,000 heart attacks that occur each year, most of them could be prevented by drastically lowering the cholesterol in your diet. This is typical of government science -- they use statistics grossly distorting the facts.

Nearly 36 percent of heart attacks occur in people over the age of 80, which could hardly be called "premature deaths." Of the 350,000 cases that are left, about half are due to unknown or unchangeable risk factors such as heredity. Thus, only 175,000 deaths are potentially preventable by any type of public health intervention, and almost all of these could be prevented simply by not smoking cigarettes.

So when a Harvard nutritionist advises you to drink a cup of corn oil every week, tell him to stick it in his crankcase.

More About Veggie Oil

Using these vegetable oils in your salad is bad enough, but when heated they are really murder. Studies have been done comparing the effect of heated vegetable oils and heated butter on the health of experimental animals. The animals fed the heated oils developed diarrhea and their fur got scruffy. All of them developed tumors and all but one died within 40 months. There were no tumors among the butter-fed group and they all lived a normal life.

Heated vegetable oil fed to animals has been shown to cause a 127 percent increase in breast cancer and Dr. David Kritchevsky of the Wistar Institute in Pennsylvania reported that vegetable oils, when fed to animals, increase rather than reduce hardening of the arteries. Some couples can't conceive because the husband isn't fertile enough. In some cases this could be due to a heavy intake of vegetable oils, as recommended by their doctor. And their doctor is simply following the guidelines of the AHA, which is committed to the heart/cholesterol hypothesis no matter what the evidence shows. What the evidence reveals is that heated vegetable oils cause testicular damage due to an absorption of the oils into the testicles.

These same vegetable oils also cause premature aging in millions of Americans. A plastic surgeon did a study in which he examined the diets of his patients and correlated them with facial skin wrinkling. Those patients eating a high vegetable fat diet had 78 percent more facial wrinkles and many appeared 20 years older than they were.

The Food and Drug Administration (FDA) occasionally grumbles about the false and misleading advertising by the vegetable oil producers. It is common knowledge among scientists that the claims for a cholesterol-lowering effect by "polyunsaturates" are simply not true and there is strong evidence that they are a menace to health. But the FDA does nothing to stop these phony and dangerous health claims. Why do you suppose the FDA looks the other way when the oil salesmen make outlandish statements that would land a vitamin promoter in jail?

The answer is simple. The chief prosecutor for the FDA resigns and where does he go? He becomes the president of the Institute of Shortening and Edible Oils! (Do you suppose that's why he couldn't get around to prosecuting the false claims of the "edible" oil industry?) It gets even smellier. At the same time, the gent who had been the legal representative for the oil boys, i.e., the man opposing the now-president of the oil institute, becomes the chief prosecutor for the FDA! I have more equally disgusting examples of your EDA at work but maybe you're getting sick. I know I am.

I can't resist telling you about one more particularly obnoxious worm: former Senator George McGovern. McGovern was simply a trollop for the vegetable oil industry. In July 1971, he announced that he would hold hearings on the "relation of diet to heart disease" and it was stated that he would only listen to the testimony of those who had already declared themselves on the side of vegetable oils. Other opinions were not requested or welcome. If you have a heart attack, send the hospital bill to McGovern.

Vegetable oils are used to manufacture that non-food called margarine. It will kill experimental animals and it will kill you, too, it just takes a little longer. If you want the whole story on the titanic grease war that was waged between the farmers (butter) and the food industry (oleo), read my book, *The Milk Book*.

All that is interesting history, but let me tell you about a paradoxical situation today that illustrates the utter hypocrisy of your government. American farmers get a whopping 70 cents a pound from the government for butter that the American consumer never sees. Because of all the anti-butter propaganda, people just aren't buying butter. Why should they? If butter is going to kill you, and margarine, a "heart food," is cheaper, then who needs butter? This same government that discourages the consumption of demon butter in the U.S., sells it by the millions of pounds to European countries, where it doesn't cause doctors and nutritionists to recoil in horror. They buy it at a cut-rate price of 50 cents a pound while we eat the imitation stuff -- and the American taxpayer makes up the difference. The Europeans must think we're nuts.

I remember, back in the late 1930s, my mother couldn't afford butter, so she bought "oleo." It came with a packet of dye that you mixed with the oleomargarine to make it look like butter. The present day increase in cancer and cardiovascular disease correlates better with the dramatic increase in the use of these saturated (hydrogenated) vegetable oils than any other dietary change. In fact, there was no other dramatic dietary change at the time.

The widespread use of the solidified vegetable oils (margarine) is nothing more than a de facto experiment on the American people without their informed consent -- and the experiment is going badly. With remarkable prescience, D.E. Salmon, chief of the Bureau of Animal Industry, said 40 years ago that an invention like oleomargarine "which introduces a radical change to the manufacture of an article of food which goes on the table of every family in the land, might produce an unexpected and remarkable effect on the public health." How right he was, but butter is getting the blame.

Scammery

The American Heart Association was singing a different tune on cholesterol a few years ago: "An immense effort has been devoted to the reduction of cholesterol levels in the blood by diet and by drugs and it must now be concluded that these efforts have had no detectable influence on the course and development of coronary heart disease." The British journal, the *Lancet*, came to the same conclusion: "The results of cholesterol studies prove nothing."

So what happened to cause this complete turnaround? Pressure from the food companies and the drug companies who pay the bills of the medical establishment -- it's called going with the buck.

As a layman, you don't get the opportunity to hear what qualified scientists are saying about this colossal scam (that's why you hired me). Dr. Hyman Engleberg, for instance, is a charter member of the Council on Atherosclerosis of the American Heart Association and here is what he has to say about the cholesterol hysteria in this country:

> Advocating strict low-fat, low-cholesterol diets for a large portion of the total American population implies that no harm can be done. This is not true.... The publicity about cholesterol has created wide-spread fear about eating, and this cannot be healthful.
>
> In many women, a cholesterol-lowering diet does lower the total cholesterol, but

decreases the high-density ... cholesterol ... to a greater extent. This is harmful and just measuring the total cholesterol gives a false sense of security.

Many eminent authorities disagree with the position of the... American Heart Association. The public has not been told about this.

Dr. Meyer Texon, Associate Professor of Forensic Medicine at New York University, has this to say:

Critical analysis of the 1982 diet statement (of the NIH) found it not to be a logical explanation of dietary recommendations, but an assemblage of obsolete and misquoted references. Major studies have shown virtually no effect of diet on serum cholesterol levels... It has been pointed out that lowering serum cholesterol by dietary modifications is open to serious question because most serum cholesterol is produced (in the body) and production increases when dietary intake is reduced. There is no correlation between either diet or blood cholesterol levels and severity of atherosclerosis ... Atherosclerosis ... occurs without relation in a causative sense to the level of cholesterol ... The experience of every practicing physician includes patients with blood lipids (fat) at any and all levels who have developed coronary atherosclerosis...

The calculated increase in life expectancy from a lifelong dietary program to reduce serum cholesterol levels ... is between three

days and three months for persons allegedly at
low risk!

The time has come to change course and to
place the cholesterol-heart disease hypothesis
in a holding pattern while more promising
alternative directions ... are explored.

Chapter 3

Count Your Eggs

E ggs are getting the most heat from the anti-cholesterol crowd. But did you hear about the elderly gentleman in the nursing home who was eating 30 eggs a day? The doctors checked his cholesterol level and it was perfectly normal (150). Examination revealed no evidence of hardening of the arteries -- and the gentleman is 88 years old!

This egg-lover had been ingesting 6,000 mg of cholesterol daily, which is 5,700 mg. more than the "recommended" amount, and had been doing this for 15 years. The investigators checked his HDL (the good cholesterol) and his LDL (the bad cholesterol) and the ratio of the two was right where the experts say it should be.

The scientists tried to explain these findings away by saying that the old gentleman had some sort of

built-in protective mechanism that enabled him to
avoid the terrible effects of Demon Cholesterol. But, as
we have explained to you, everyone, except a tiny
minority of people with a congenital defect in their
cholesterol metabolism, has this built-in cholesterol-
regulating system.

They just couldn't leave the old guy alone. A
psychiatrist and a clinical psychologist tried to alter
his eating habits which they called "compulsive
behavior." They admitted to failure which brings up
some interesting questions: (1) Is the old man smarter
on nutritional matters than the doctors? After all, he is
a healthy 88. (2) Is it possible that the massive
cholesterol intake has actually protected the old gent
from the ravages of modern life? Yes, it's possible.

The AMA's latest propaganda missile for the
meat-eating public is a report called the "AMA Fat/
Cholesterol Education Program." The first paragraph
of this "educational tool", as they call it, contains an
error that sets the tone for the entire apocryphal piece:
"Your risk of developing atherosclerosis and coronary
heart disease... is directly related to the amount of
cholesterol in your blood." For the ample reasons we
have given you in this treatise, you know that simply
is not a scientifically proven fact.

This is followed by an equally untrue statement:
"The risk can be reduced by making changes that
lower the cholesterol level." And then piffle that is
even worse: "Lowering your cholesterol by 15 percent

would reduce your risk of heart attack by 30 percent." Too bad it's not that easy. Lower it 50 percent and maybe you'll have a massive stroke and then you will never have to worry again about a heart attack.

And this one really makes me wince: "Most people can lower their cholesterol levels ... by reducing their dietary intake of cholesterol and fat." Offal, effluvium, and scientific bosh. Cholesterol and animal fat may actually lower your cholesterol (and you will enjoy some great meals).

The AMA's National Cholesterol Education Program is now recommending that all adults over the age of 20 be screened for high blood cholesterol. Can you imagine how many barrels of bucks this will put into the hands of doctors and their laboratories? Two doctors in New England did a study to determine how much it would cost to "treat" high cholesterol with the currently recommended methods (including the use of the toxic drugs now being used and the resulting drug side effects). They concluded that it would cost one million dollars per year per patient for each year of life saved. Are you worth a million dollars a year of someone else's money? I know the answer to that question, but is it worth paying a tax collector, a lawyer, or a psychiatrist that much? Checking cholesterol on everyone over 20, and then acting on those findings according to the paranoiac (and self-serving) delusions of the American Medical Association would bankrupt the nation.

The pamphlet also says, "The ideal time to have your blood cholesterol level measured is when you are already in your doctor's office for a routine visit." Why are you going to the doctor for a aroutine visit?" Has he become a priest or something? Stay away from your doctor as much as you can, except maybe on the golf course or the pool hall, and if he brings up that cholesterol stuff, tell him to read this report and then ask him what he is doing about his cholesterol.

Of course, this AMA "education" pamphlet wasn't written by doctors. The only thing doctors know about nutrition is that it wasn't very important until an addlepated scientist did some cholesterol experiments on rabbits (which he bungled) and cholesterol was thus changed from an essential nutrient to something akin to botulism. Want to know who wrote this puffery? Here's a hint from the pamphlet, *Tips on Eating for a Healthier Heart:* "Corn oil margarines provide the perfect alternative to more saturated fats like butter," and "Egg substitutes provide the perfect alternative to whole eggs." The sponsors of this blitz against normal food are Fleischmann's "100 percent corn oil" margarine and EggBeaters, both of which are subsidiaries of Nabisco, the nation's largest purveyor of junk food. The last page of the pamphlet has two convenient coupons so that you can order your start-up supply of plastic butter and eggless eggs. There is also a coupon for Art Ulene's video, "Count Out Cholesterol," which is more of the same bad nutritional advice.

"Where's the Beef?"

The food persecuted most, after eggs, is red meat. What is meant by "red meat" is beef, lamb, and pork. It is curious the way specialties of science will set aside large bodies of information that relate in an important way to their area of science and pretend that they don't exist. It's human nature. There is no other way to explain it. A jaded scientist once said, "An 'academic discipline' is a group of scholars who have agreed not to ask certain embarrassing questions about key assumptions." The present rush to vegetarianism is a classic example. There is little doubt that the shift to a basic vegetable diet from one of meat, meat products, and wild fruit was a health disaster for mankind, we are told the very opposite by today's experts in nutrition.

The idea that these meats are bad for you is, if you'll pardon the expression, baloney. If you want to stay healthy, I recommend that you *include a good portion of red meat in your diet.* Believe me, the media and many doctors serve more baloney than scientific facts.

Red meat is by far your best source of high-quality protein in the best balance for human consumption. It contains iron, amino acids, B-12, vitamins A and D, zinc, calcium, and, if you leave the fat where it belongs (on the meat), cholesterol. The mental and physical development of children depends on a proper balance of all the nutrients, and no amount of vegetable or other protein provides this ideal combination, in the right proportions, like red meat.

The present staples of civilization, tubers and cereals, are poor sources of everything but energy. They weren't chosen for their food value, but because they have a long shelf life and a prolific growth rate. Compared to meat, they are poor in protein, vitamins, and minerals.

Even when vegetables contain the required minerals for good health, they are often useless to man because of certain chemical bonding. The chemical group called phytates form chemical bonds with the minerals in the human intestinal tract making them insoluble and unable to pass across the intestinal lining. Thus, instead of enriching your body, you are enriching the local waste disposal plant. Iron, zinc, and calcium are all difficult to get in proper amounts from a vegetarian diet, especially a diet based on wheat or corn. Oxalates and phosphates, common in cereals and tubers such as potatoes, also inhibit iron absorption. Iron deficiency anemia may result if the diet is focused on these foods.

A diet fit for a zebra can be a serious handicap if strictly adhered to. Corn is poor in the essential amino acids, lysine, and tryptophan and is a poor source of iron and niacin (B-3). In fact, corn contains an anti-niacin substance which increases the requirement for niacin in the face of a deficiency due to the corn diet itself! In the serious vegetarian, this is a sure road to pellagra. A similar situation can develop with a diet composed primarily of rice. The rice has a poor protein content which inhibits the activity of vitamin A. Deficiency in vitamin A leads to skin diseases, intestinal diseases, and, if severe, blindness. A heavy rice diet can also lead to a thiamine (B-1) deficiency called beriberi.

America's hospitals are full of people with beriberi, pellagra, scurvy, iron-deficiency anemia, hypovitaminosis-A, mineral deficiencies, kwashiakor, and other deficiency diseases, but they are almost always overlooked because they are not as gross, and thus as obvious, as those same conditions seen in Third World countries. A little meat in the diet, especially if it is cooked rare, will clear up every single one of these conditions. For man, there is nothing "natural" about a pure vegetable/fruit diet. It's hard to make it on a diet intended for rodents and you can forget about the Olympics, Wimbledon, and the Super Bowl because you're not going to beat the cut.

Dr. Weston Price, in his monumental studies in the South Pacific, demonstrated that when islanders abandoned their high-protein fish diets their facial configurations changed, with the face becoming narrower and the jaws no longer able to properly accommodate the teeth. The slight overbite that we consider normal with our teeth is a pathological condition and not normal at all. It developed, as proven by ancient skeletons, as a result of the dietary shift away from a primarily meat diet to one of tubers and grain.

Incidentally, my Grandma Bell never got fat eating all that fat; she never weighed over a 100 pounds. But I bet your doctor never told you that eating fat doesn't make you fat. Eating too much sugar, starch, and fat makes you fat, but eating fat alone won't do it. In fact, I've seen patients lose 50 pounds on a strict meat and fat diet.

But if you don't eat beef, lamb, or pork for "philosophical" reasons, at least be a fishatarian. That way you will get some decent protein and animal fat. (I don't know why some people just can't stand the idea of a lamb being killed for food -- he would never have had any life at all but for being grown as food. But a suffering fish doesn't bother them aphilosophically." It's downright racist if you ask me -- don't fish have feelings?)

Let me tell you about the !Kung San tribe of Botswana. (I don't know why they put the "!" in the spelling of their tribe. It's there and that's all I can tell you.) These people eat a diet that contains 24 percent hunted meat. They have never heard of Oreo cookies, TCBY, Captain Crunch, lite this and lite that, or any of the other plastic foods that we consume, and they think you are nuts for not eating a good steak two or three times a week, since you can afford it. They said to me that Western man should bury his spear -- what good is it to him? A very good question.

And as for those greenies who want to go back to nature, why don't they really go back to nature and start eating meat? Studies on the !Kung San (also the Dobe! Kung and the / /Gana San -- those are not misprints) have shown that they have a nutritional status comparable to the upper classes of our most advanced countries. In fact the !Kung exceeded recommended dietary standards for all minerals and vitamins. Why? Because they eat meat, that's why. And they have no diabetes, hypertension, cavities, heart disease, hemorrhoids, varicose veins, hiatal hernia, or decline in hearing or eyesight with advancing age.

The Nata San are a different story. They tend to hang around the white man's cattle stations, so they have laid down their spears and eaten his food. As would be expected, they are subject to all the deficiency diseases seen in poor Third World countries. And the Hadza tribe, which lived on the rich African savanna, was never known to go hungry until they were persuaded to live on reservations like American Indians. Then the tribes' people began to suffer from hunger when the food truck didn't show up. Isn't that a subtle form of slavery?

We need to revise our thinking and realize that a low-meat, low-cholesterol, low-animal-fat diet is not synonymous with good science and good nutrition. The paleontological data simply doesn't support it. We tend to measure our progress based on comparisons with the conditions of the 14th to the

18th centuries. But we are comparing ourselves with the most impoverished, the most disease-ridden, and the shortest-lived populations in recorded human history -- anything would be an improvement. You can't extrapolate back from there and assume that things were always that bad, because they weren't. Things were pretty good until the agricultural revolution.

Clearly, modern agriculture provides more people with the means of at least staying alive, but let's not confuse a diet of wheat, rice, or corn with good nutrition. Realistically, there simply isn't enough room or natural food resources for all of us to revert to some modified form of hunting and gathering, no matter how beneficial that would be for mankind. But man's ingenuity must be directed toward developing some form of animal protein that will be nutritious, cheap, and readily available. The answer is there, it's all around us, but few people who worry about these things seem to have noticed. The answer is insects.

It seems that everything on earth was put here for a reason and insects weren't put here just to feed birds and ruin picnics. A large variety of insects are plentiful, nutritious, and even delicious: the Ugandan grasshopper, for example.

But while the world is grappling with mal-nutrition and starvation, there is no reason why you should eat like a Bangladeshi in a land overflowing with milk, cheese, butter, and beautifully marbled steaks. At least that's what my friends the !Kung San say. Loosen up and remember the words of Admiral Farragot at Manila Bay in 1864: "Damn the tortillas -- full speed ahead!"

Dr. Robert Atkins, author *of Nutritional Breakthrough,* summed up the situation quite nicely. Dr. Atkins is often asked by the media, "Why do you allow eggs and saturated fats? Aren't you worried about raising your patients' cholesterol and creating heart disease?" His reply: "I've observed thousands of patients on all sorts of diets, and those who ate eggs and meat and cheese did very well *in all respects.* If anything, their heart disease improved."

Commonly Consumed Protein

Sources*	Saturated Fat (g)	Calories	Cholesterol (mg)	Fat (g)
Chicken breast (skin on, fried)	11.2	221	72	3.0
Chicken thigh (skinless, roasted)	9.3	178	81	2.6
Beef flank (broiled)	8.6	176	57	3.7
Pork loin chop (bone in, broiled)	6.9	165	70	2.5
Leg of lamb (roasted)	6.6	162	78	2.3

*Based on one cooked serving.

Turkey dark meat (skinless, roasted)	6.1	159	72	2.1
Chicken breast (skinless, roasted)	3.0	140	72	0.9
Turkey light meat (skinless, roasted)	2.7	133	59	0.9
Flounder (dry-heat cooked)	1.3	99	58	0.3

Sources: "A Nationwide Survey of the Composition and Marketing of Pork Products at Retail," University of Wisconsin, 1990: USDA handbooks 8-5, 8-13, and 8-17.

The Chicken Scoop

For some reason, chicken has avoided the cholesterol and fat rap. But if you study the table above, you'll see that chicken has more cholesterol than pork, beef, or lamb, even if the skin has been removed. When I ask patients, "Do you eat any meat?" They invariably reply, "No, I'm a vegetarian (pause), I do eat a little chicken every week." I guess they eat chicken and avoid a good steak because the chicken meat is white and so it must be cleaner than beef or pork. I can assure you that nothing could be further from the truth. A chicken will poop anywhere and then turn around and eat it. A pig won't poop in his parlor -- they're clean when given a chance.

Chapter 4

A Bit of History

Periodically, America goes through an anti-meat, anti-fat crusade. In 1926, a small but vociferous group proclaimed that meat and fat caused kidney disease, arthritis, and high blood pressure. Part of this may have been the continuing concept that anything as good-tasting as meat and fat must be bad for you. Sixty-eight years later, the anti-meat doomsayers are at it again. But this time they have the doctors, the government, the legalized drug pushers of the pharmaceutical industry, and the hustlers from the vegetable oil industry on their side -- the cow, the pig, and the egg-laying chicken are in for some hard times -- it's not going to help the poor struggling farmer either.

There is a vast difference between what dieticians and many nutritionists tell us and what paleonutrition, derived from scientific paleopathology (the study of disease in ancient peoples) has conclusively proven. The accepted "science" today is that cholesterol causes hardening of the arteries and animal fat does the same, along with causing a myriad of other diseases including hypertension, bowel cancer, breast cancer, obesity, etc. The fact that the scientific literature proves nothing of the sort does not slow down the American Heart Association or the hucksters on your television.

Studies on ancient hunter/gatherer tribes, using primarily bone and teeth remains, indicate that they fared relatively well and worked relatively little. When man moved to an agricultural, primarily vegetarian diet, he began deteriorating with a decrease in stature, an increase in nutritional deficiencies, and the beginning of the diseases of modern man, including tuberculosis, arthritis, dental caries (rotting teeth), and cancer. The present attitudes on nutrition are based on a narrow view of man's history, primarily of Western society, and ignore the extensive findings of paleontologists to whom American dieticians and nutritionists don't speak. And of whom, in fact, they have probably never heard.

Monkey Business

If you think man ascended from the ape, then there is further proof that humans have always been carnivorous. It has always been assumed that our "ancestors," the primates, are vegetarians. However, Jane Goodall studied apes in their natural habitat and discovered that they eat meat on a regular basis. Baboons eat vervet monkeys and other small animals. Chimps eat small baboons.

The National Zoo in Washington, D.C. attempted to breed Amazonian monkeys. They were feeding them a total fruit diet and, although a lot of monkey business went on, there were no pregnancies. Within weeks of feeding them meat, pregnancies began to occur.

Dr. H. Leon Abrams, an anthropologist, says that man has been almost exclusively a meat-eater for 99 percent of the time he has been on earth. So, don't believe that stuff about man being a natural vegetarian. The Australopithecenes would laugh in your face.

If you fall for the propaganda of the American Heart Association and the vegetable oil hustlers and go strictly vegetarian, here's what you can expect: an increase in cavities, a B-12 deficiency, a folic acid deficiency, an increase in the likelihood of contracting leukemia, osteoporosis, amino acid deficiency-- and you will look like death warmed over. (I can spot a flaming vegetarian a block away.)

They did a study at Hebrew University in Israel on 119 strict vegetarians and found that all of them were amino acid-deficient. If babies are fed a strict vegetarian diet, they do not grow at a normal rate.

They get shortchanged on B-12, folic acid, zinc, calories, proteins, calcium, and riboflavin (B-2). Even a breast-fed baby may become malnourished if the mother has been a true vegetarian (no meat, fish, milk, butter, eggs, etc.) for a number of years.

Icelanders have cavities just like people in other modern societies, but it didn't used to be that way. The director of the National Museum in Iceland reports the paleolithic record shows that for the 600 years between 1200 and 1800, Icelanders had no dental cavities. They lived on milk and milk products, mutton, beef, and fish. They had no fruits and vegetables and no carbohydrates.

The Pueblo Indians worship the corn god, but he has not been grateful. They subsist on corn, squash, and beans and have the most wretched teeth of all the American Indians.

Living off the Fat of the Land in Africa

The lifestyles of many tribes in Africa completely refute the cholesterol theories of today's dieticians (who simply believe what the American Heart Association tells them). The Samburu tribe of northern Kenya continues to baffle the cholesterol experts. The average American, with his hardened arteries, eats a meager 80 grams of fat per day. The Samburu eats 400 grams of fat per day and has a normal cholesterol level.

The Masai to the south eats a 60 percent saturated fat diet and has never heard of Mazola or EggBeaters. They have very little heart disease, consistently normal blood pressure, no obesity, and a complete absence of rheumatoid arthritis. degenerative arthritis, and gout. The average Samburu or Masai child has a cholesterol value of 138. The average American child, 202. With increasing age, the native cholesterol values go down and the American values go up. Beyond the age of 55, the mean cholesterol value of the African is 122. The mean cholesterol value for American men of this age is 234.

The Karimejong tribesmen of Uganda, as the Masai and Samburu, live entirely on the products of their cattle, and so eat nothing but meat, animal fat, milk, and blood. They are extremely healthy (fierce, too) and are not subject to the diseases of the 20th century such as heart disease, cancer, and arthritis.

Dr. George Mann, who did much of the African research, said: "The studies show no support for the contention that a large intake of dairy fat and meat necessarily causes either hypercholesterolemia or coronary heart disease... The hypothesis relating saturated animal fat to the causation of hyper-cholesterolemia and cardiovascular disease remains dubious. We favor the conclusion that diet fat is not responsible for coronary disease." (The Samburu don't get cholesterol gall stones either.)

Studies on non-industrial societies all reflect a preference for animal protein. The Tasmanians have an unusual taboo; they don't eat fish. But they love crabs and other shellfish. (A taboo against shellfish has developed in the U.S. -- leaving more for me.) The Tasmanians also like ants, grubworms, snake, lizard, kangaroo, wallaby, bandicoot (I don't know what it is, either), and the succulent wombat.

On the Andaman Islands, which are located precisely in the middle of nowhere, the people relish cat, lizards, snakes, rats, dugong, mollusks, and turtles. The Jivaro of the Amazon eat ant larvae because, they say, the fat is good for them. How can people without any schooling whatsoever, who have never heard of Jane Brody, the *New York Times* health expert, know that? (Jane wouldn't approve, so they must be reading my material.)

The Aztecs ate ants, mosquito eggs, toasted grasshoppers, worms -- and each other. The "each other" thing was a religious deal -- the priests always got the best parts.

The list of peoples who live almost entirely on animal food with little or no fruits or vegetables is voluminous. The Kazaks of central Asia, the Todas of southern India, the Nuer of East Africa, the Tierra del Fuegans of South America, and others I have enumerated in this report, don't care a fig about "the basic food groups" and they don't die of the things we die of: heart attack, stroke, and cancer. They die of infection, trauma (it's a jungle out there), or old age.

The paleopathologists, to whom no one pays the slightest attention, can tell you a lot about how man should eat. They know what humans have been eating for thousands of years. They aren't selling "fat-free" hamburgers, electrocardiograms, cholesterol tests, anti-cholesterol drugs, cholesterol-free oils, or any other of the accoutrements of the cholesterol scam. They just report the scientific findings on what man has been eating for thousands of years. But there is no communication between these scientists and the dieticians of the American Heart Association -they've never *heard* of a paleopathologist.

It's amazing what these scientists can tell us about the nutrition and eating habits of ancient man from studying their skeletal remains. A condition called porotic osteoporosis has proven to be a valuable marker for disease consequent to poor nutrition. Most researchers in the field agree with professor Alan H. Goodman of the University of Massachusetts, who noted that as groups change from a hunting-gathering economy to one based fully on agriculture, the incidence of infectious diseases increases dramatically.

This has been confirmed by many others. J. Lawrence Angel of the Department of Anthropology, National Museum of Natural History, states that "nutrition became progressively... poorer with early farming. This applied especially to protein from red meat needed for adequate childhood growth... An increase in disease was also involved."

Dr. Kenneth A.R. Kennedy of the Department of Anthropology, Cornell University, reported on paleodemographic studies in South Asia: "The adoption of intensified utilization and processing of vegetable food sources that allowed for greater food stability led to lower quality nutrition and increase in certain pathologies... These pathological variables are represented in skeletal remains by higher incidences of porotic hyperostosis, caries (cavities), abscess, long bone deformations, rickets, and scurvy." He also noted a decrease in stature and shorter life span when a shift was made from a primarily meat diet to a meat-deficient farm diet. Exactly the same conclusion was drawn from a study done by Northern Illinois University, on the aboriginals of primitive Georgia.

And now even Jane Brody, the health expert from the *New York Times* we discussed earlier, is beginning to see the light. She reported in the August 24, 1994 issue of the Times, "Just when consumers think they have mastered the connections between dietary fats, cholesterol, and heart disease, another finding emerges to confuse the issue.... Now researchers from the Boston University School of Medicine say that all this advice is off base and will not adequately reduce the risk of fat-clogged arteries that lead to heart attacks and strokes. Rather, their preliminary studies indicate, a very low-fat diet may in itself touch off heart disease."

So you can see that there is a wealth of proof that you do not have to take the anti-cholesterol warriors and propagandists seriously. Eat all the meat you want (with the fat on it), use real cream in your coffee, not "creamer" (a combination of sugar and vegetable oil), and slather real butter on your morning toast -- it will go well with your three-egg omelet. If you follow this dietary advice, you'll probably make your three score and ten -- if you do everything else right.

Action to Take

(1)   Get a reasonable amount of meat and fat in your diet.

(2)   Avoid low-cholesterol foods and all type of fake food. That includes anything marked "lite," "cholesterol-free," or "recommended by the American Heart Association." Look at all the products you buy on a regular basis and stop using any that have highly saturated vegetable oils in the ingredients. That would include most processed cookies, cakes, and candies.

(3)   Avoid all vegetable oils except olive oil and linseed oil.

(4)   Butter or lard should be used when cooking -- look hard to find the lard. (It's behind the Crisco.)

(5)   Cut out all sugar and sugar substitutes.

(6)   Walk two miles a day.

(7) When it comes to cholesterol, remember that your weight is usually irrelevant.

(8) Avoid artificial milk -- that includes homogenized, pasteurized, vitamin A and D, skim, lowfat, and other dairy abominations. The only place you can legally buy fresh, natural, "raw" milk is from a farm. If you can't get it straight from the cow, don't drink it.

If you can't get milk from the farm and you refuse to stop drinking milk, I may have a solution. It's not perfect, but it's a great improvement over the chalky-white and sometimes chalky-tasting stuff at the dairy counter. Buy skim milk and some whipping cream. Skim milk is homogenized, but there is so little fat present that the amount of xanthine oxidase you are exposed to is negligible. The whipping cream is heavy enough that homogenization isn't necessary. It is pasteurized, but otherwise it's a pretty good product.

Mix the skim milk and cream, four parts skim and one part whipping cream. If it's too rich or too thin, you can vary it to your liking. When you first try this on your cereal, you will be amazed at the improvement.

(9) Stay away from margarine, oleo, and any other butter or fat substitutes. That includes Pam, Crisco, and other shortenings.

(10) Avoid tap water. It contains chlorine, fluorine, and aluminum. Either buy a filter that takes out

all of these contaminants, or buy spring water. Contact the company you buy from and ask for a report on their company and a list of ingredients in their water.

11) Get plenty of sunshine without sunglasses or heavy sunscreen.

(12) Make sure that you breast feed your babies. Also, don't forget to tell your friends and loved ones that baby formulas are the worst thing they can feed their babies.

(13) Get your friends and community leaders to read 7he Milk Book. Included in this book is information on how you can order your copy of this important book.

(14) Stop smoking, or forget all of the above.

Suggested Further Reading

Periodicals

American Journal of Public Health, May 16, 1994.

New England Journal of Medicine, January 10, 1991, pp.121-123.

New England Journal of Medicine, December 19, 1991, p.1812.

Patient Care, February 28, 1989, p.8.

Grand Rapids (Michigan) Press, August 16, 1990, (AP) Front page article on margarine.

The Cutting Edge, December 1987.

The Journal of the American Geriatrics Society, August 1969, p.727.

The Wall Street Journal, June 14, 1988, p.1.

The Wall Street Journal, October 6,1987, front page, second section.

New Scientist, May 19, 1990, pp. 38-41.

U.S. News and World Report, October 19, 1987, pp. 68-69.

Journal of the American Medical Association, November 28, 1986, pp. 2867-2870.

Internal Medicine News, Vol. 20, #12, p. 15 (Eggs).

AMA News, December 11, 1987, p. 3 (The Cholesterol Propaganda Blitz).

Medical Tribune, October 7, 1987, p. 3.

Hippocrates, May/June 1990, pp. 37-43, July-August 1987, pp. 16-19 (olive oil).

Books

The Cholesterol Controversy, Pinckney and Pinckney, Sherbourne Press, 1973, Los Angeles.

Health and the Rise of Civilization, Cohen, Yale University Press, 1989.

Cannibals and Kings, Harris, Random House, 1977.

The Paleolithic Prescription, Eaton, Harper and Row, 1988.

Food and Evolution, Harris and Ross, Temple University Press, 1987.

Paleopathology at the Origins of Agriculture, Cohen and Armelagos, Academic Press, 1984.

Other

Mr. Wayne Martin, 25 Orchard Drive, Fairhope, Alabama 36532, has an encyclopedic knowledge of the cholesterol literature and is generous in sharing his knowledge. This gentleman is not a doctor. I do not mention that as a derogation, but as a positive qualification. His mind is not closed.

Index

A

!Kung, 46, 47, 49
!Kung San, 46, 47, 49
//Gana San, 47
Abrams, Dr . H. Leon, 53
Alcohol,10
Aluminum, 2, 60
American Heart
        Association, 12, 13,
        25, 26, 29-31, 33, 36,
        37, 52-54, 57, 59
American Indians, 47, 54
American Medical
        Association, 1, 5, 6,
        8, 16, 24, 40-42, 64
Amino acids ,43, 44
Andaman Islands, 56
Angel, J. Lawrence, 57
Anitchkow, Dr., 11
Arthritis, 51, 52, 55
Aspirin, 9
Associated Press, 23

Atherosclerosis, 3, 7, 11,
        17, 26, 36-37, 40
Atkins, Dr. Robert, 49
Australopithecenes, 53
Aztecs, 56

B

Bendett, Dr. Earl P., 17
Beriberi, 45
Blindness, 45
Boston University School
        of Medicine, 58
Botswana, 46
Bristol-Myers,10
Brody, Jane, 56, 58
Bureau of Animal
        Industry, 20, 35
Butter, 1, 2, 7, 18-21, 24,
        26, 27, 31, 32, 34-36,
        42, 48, 54, 59, 60
Butyric acid (butyrate), 21, 25,
        27, 32, 33, 52, 55, 56

C

Calcium, 43, 44, 54
Cancer, 7, 17, 18, 21, 25
           27, 32, 33, 52, 55, 56
Captain Crunch, 46
Caster, Dr. W.O., 25
Cavities, 47, 53, 54, 58
Cheese, 2, 48, 49
Chemotherapy,16
Chlorine, 60
Cholesterol 1-3, 5-19, 21,
           24-31, 33, 36-43, 47,
           49, 50, 52, 54, 55,
           57-59, 64,65
Colestid, 18
Corn oil, 3, 16, 22, 25,
           27, 32, 42
Cornell University,58
Council on Atherosclerosis
           (AHA), 36

D

De Gaulle,Charles, 2
Diabetes, 11, 47
Diarrhea, 32
Dobe !Kung, 47
Duck fat, 2

E

East Africa, 10, 56
Eggs, 2, 3, 16, 39, 42, 51, 59
EggBeaters, 3, 42, 55
Engleberg, Dr. Hyman, 36

F

Fish, 7, 30, 45, 46, 54, 56
Fleischmann's, 3, 42
Fluoride, 2
Fluorine, 60
Folic acid, 53, 54
Food and Drug Administration
           (FDA),11, 33,34

G

Goodall, Jane, 53
Goodman, Alan H., 57
Grandma Bell, 25, 46
Gullickson, Dr. T. W., 22

H

Hadza tribe, 47
Halperin, Dr. Alan K., 13
Harmon, Dr. Denham, 31
Harvard University,10,
           23, 25, 26, 28, 29, 32
HDL cholesterol, 24, 39
Heart attack, 3, 8, 16, 27,
           34, 41, 56
Heart disease, 2, 5, 7, 8, 10
           18, 23, 25, 27-29, 34
           36, 38, 40, 47, 49, 55, 58
Hebrew University, 53
Hemorrhoids, 47
Hiatal hernia, 47
Hyper-cholesterolemia, 16
Hypertension, 11, 47, 52
Hypocholesterolemia, 7
Hypovitarninosis-A, 45

I

International Lipid
  Information Bureau
  (LIB),12
Irish Brothers Study, 26
Iron, 7, 43-45
Iron-deficiency anemia, 45

J

Jackson, Jerry, 7

K

Kazaks of central Asia, 56
Kennedy, Dr.Kenneth
  A.R., 57
Kritchevsky,Dr.David, 32
Kwashiakor, 45

L

LaFollette,Senator
  "Fighting Bob," 20
Lancet, 17, 36
LDL cholesterol, 24, 39
Leukemia, 29, 53
Linseed oil, 25
Lopid, 11, 18
Lysine, 44

M

Madison Avenue, 25
Mann,Dr.George, 27-29, 55
Margarine, 3, 18-27, 34,
  35, 42, 60, 63
Masai, 55

Mazola, 25, 55
McGovern, George, 34
McNarnara, Dr. Donald,
  15-17
Merck,Sharp &Dohme
  (MSD), 7, 8, 10, 13
Mevacor, 8, 18
Milk, 5, 7, 22, 28, 30, 34,
  48, 54, 55, 60, 61
Mineral deficiencies, 45

N

Nabisco, 25, 42
Nata San, 47
National Cholesterol
  Education Program,
  40, 41
National Heart,Lung,and
  Blood Institute
  (NHLBI), 8, 12, 13, 31
National Institutes of
  Health, 29
National Museum in
  Iceland, 54
National Zoo in Washington,
  D.C., 53
New England Journal of
  Medicine (NEJM), 9,
  10, 12, 63
New York Times, 56, 58
New York University, 37
Niacin (B-3), 44
Northern Illinois
  University, 58

Nuer of East Africa, 56
Nutritional Breakthrough, 49

O

Oleomargarine (oleo), 21,
    34, 35, 60
Olive oil, 25, 26, 59, 64
Olympics, 45
Oreo cookies, 46
Osteoporosis, 18, 53, 57
Oxalates, 44

P

Pellagra, 45
Phosphates, 44
Polyunsaturated fats, 26
Premature aging, 3, 33
Price,Dr.Weston ,45
Pritikin, 29
Pueblo Indians, 54
Purdue University, 17

Q

Questran, 18

R

Red meat, 7, 27, 31, 43,44, 57
Riboflavin (B-2), 54
Rockefeller University, 15

S

Salmon,D.E. ,20, 35
Samburu, 10, 54, 55
Scurvy, 45, 58

Shoney's, 19
Southwestern Medical
    School,11
Stare, Fred, 26-30
Story, Dr. John, 17
Stroke, 3, 41, 56
Super Bowl, 45

T

Tasmanians, 55, 56
TCBY, 46
Texon, Dr. Meyer, 37
The Milk Book, 5, 34, 61
Tierra del Fuegans of
    South America, 56
Tips On Eating for a
    Healthier Heart, 42
Todas of southern India, 56
Tryptophan, 44

U

U.S. Bureau of Animal
    Industry, 20
Udaipur, India, 18
Ugandan grasshopper, 48
Ulene, Art, 42
United States Dairy
    Association (USDA), 50
University of Georgia, 25
University of Massachusetts,
    57
University of Minnesota, 22,27
University of Nebraska
    School of Medicine, 31

University of Washington, 17
University of Wisconsin, 50
Upjohn, 10

V

Varicose veins, 47
Vegetable oil, 18, 22, 23,
    26, 31-34, 51, 53, 59
Veterans Administration
    Medical Center in
    Albuquerque, New
    Mexico, 13
Vitamin A, 45, 60
Vitamin B-12, 43, 53, 54

Vitamin D,10, 20, 21, 30,
    35, 43, 53, 60

W

Walton, Bill, 18
Warner-Lambert, 11, 12
White, Dr. Paul Dudley, 30
Willett, Dr.Walter, 23
Williams, Joseph, 12
Wimbledon, 45
Wistar Institute, 32

Z

Zinc, 43, 44, 54

About Doctor William Campbell Douglass II

Dr. Douglass reveals medical truths, and deceptions, often at risk of being labeled heretical. He is consumed by a passion for living a long healthy life, and wants his readers to share that passion. Their health and well-being comes first. He is anti-dogmatic, and unwavering in his dedication to improve the quality of life of his readers. He has been called "the conscience of modern medicine," a "medical maverick," and has been voted "Doctor of the Year" by the National Health Federation. His medical experiences are far reaching-from battling malaria in Central America - to fighting deadly epidemics at his own health clinic in Africa - to flying with U.S. Navy crews as a flight surgeon - to working for 10 years in emergency medicine here in the States. These learning experiences, not to mention his keen storytelling ability and wit, make Dr. Douglass' newsletters (Daily Dose and Real Health) and books uniquely interesting and fun to read. He shares his no-frills, no-bull approach to health care, often amazing his readers by telling them to ignore many widely-hyped good-health practices (like staying away from red meat, avoiding coffee, and eating like a bird), and start living again by eating REAL food, taking some inexpensive supplements, and doing the pleasurable things that make life livable. Readers get all this, plus they learn how to burn fat, prevent cancer, boost libido, and so much more. And, Dr. Douglass is not afraid to challenge the latest studies that come out, and share the real story with his readers. Dr. William C. Douglass has led a colorful, rebellious, and crusading life. Not many physicians would dare put their professional reputations on the line as many times as this courageous healer has. A vocal opponent of "business-as-usual" medicine, Dr. Douglass has championed patients' rights and physician commitment to wellness throughout his career. This dedicated physician has repeatedly gone far beyond the call of duty in his work to spread the truth about alternative therapies. For a full year, he endured economic and physical hardship to work with physicians at the Pasteur Institute in St. Petersburg, Russia, where advanced research on photoluminescence was being conducted. Dr. Douglass comes from a distinguished family of physicians. He is the fourth generation Douglass to practice medicine, and his son is also a physician. Dr. Douglass graduated from the University of Rochester, the Miami School of Medicine, and the Naval School of Aviation and Space Medicine.

You want to protect those you love from the health dangers the authorities aren't telling you about, and learn the incredible cures that they've scorned and ignored?
Subscribe to the free Daily Dose updates "...the straight scoop about health, medicine, and politics." by sending an e-mail to real_sub@agoramail.net with the word "subscribe" in the subject line.

Dr. William Campbell Douglass'
Real Health:

Had Enough?

Enough turkey burgers and sprouts?

Enough forcing gallons of water down your throat?

Enough exercising until you can barely breathe?

Before you give up everything just because "everyone" says it's healthy...

Learn the facts from Dr. William Campbell Douglass, medicine's most acclaimed myth-buster. In every issue of Dr. Douglass' Real Health newsletter, you'll learn shocking truths about "junk medicine" and how to stay healthy while eating eggs, meat and other foods you love.

With the tips you'll receive from Real Health, you'll see your doctor less, spend a lot less money and be happier and healthier while you're at it. The road to Real Health is actually easier, cheaper and more pleasant than you dared to dream.

Subscribe to Real Health today by calling 1-800-981-7162 or visit the Real Health web site at www.realhealthnews.com.
Use promotional code : DRHBDZZZ

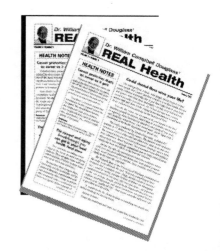

If you knew of a procedure that could save thousands, maybe millions, of people dying from AIDS, cancer, and other dreaded killers....

Would you cover it up?

It's unthinkable that what could be the best solution ever to stopping the world's killer diseases is being ignored, scorned, and rejected. But that is exactly what's happening right now.

The procedure is called "photoluminescence". It's a thoroughly tested, proven therapy that uses the healing power of the light to perform almost miraculous cures.

This remarkable treatment works its incredible cures by stimulating the body's own immune responses. That's why it cures so many ailments--and why it's been especially effective against AIDS! Yet, 50 years ago, it virtually disappeared from the halls of medicine.

Why has this incredible cure been ignored by the medical authorities of this country? You'll find the shocking answer here in the pages of this new edition of Into the Light. Now available with the blood irradiation Instrument Diagram and a complete set of instructions for building your own "Treatment Device". Also includes details on how to use this unique medical instrument.

Into the Light

Into
the
Light

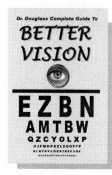

Dr. Douglass' Complete Guide to Better Vision

A report about eyesight and what can be done to improve it naturally. But I've also included information about how the eye works, brief descriptions of various common eye conditions, traditional remedies to eye problems, and a few simple suggestions that may help you maintain your eyesight for years to come.
-William Campbell Douglass II, MD

The Hypertension Report.
Say Good Bye to High Blood Pressure.

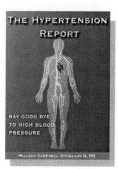

An estimated 50 million Americans have high blood pressure. Often called the "silent killer" because it may not cause symptoms until the patient has suffered serious damage to the arterial system. Diet, exercise, potassium supplements chelation therapy and practically anything but drugs is the way to go and alternatives are discussed in this report.

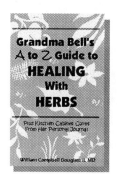

Grandma Bell's A To Z Guide To Healing With Herbs.

This book is all about - coming home. What I once believed to be old wives' tales - stories long destroyed by the new world of science - actually proved to be the best treatment for many of the common ailments you and I suffer through. So I put a few of them together in this book with the sincere hope that Grandma Bell's wisdom will help you recover your common sense, and take responsibility for your own health. -William Campbell Douglass II, MD

Prostate Problems:
Safe, Simple, Effective Relief for Men over 50.

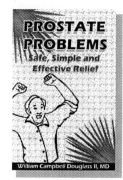

Don't be frightened into surgery or drugs you may not need. First, get the facts about prostate problems... know all your options, so you can make the best decisions. This fully documented report explains the dangers of conventional treatments, and gives you alternatives that could save you more than just money!

Color me Healthy
The Healing Powers
of Colors

"He's crazy!"
"He's got to be a quack!"
"Who gave this guy his medical license?"
"He's a nut case!"

In case you're wondering, those are the reactions you'll probably get if you show your doctor this report. I know the idea of healing many common ailments simply by exposing them to colored light sounds far-fetched, but when you see the evidence, you'll agree that color is truly an amazing medical breakthrough.

*When I first heard the stories,
I reacted much the same way.
But the evidence so
convinced me, that I had to
try color therapy in my practice.
My results were truly amazing.*

-William Campbell Douglass II, MD

Order your complete set of Roscolene filters (choice of 3 sizes) to be used with the "Color Me Healthy" therapy. The eleven Roscolene filters are # 809, 810, 818, 826, 828, 832, 859, 861, 866, 871, and 877. The filters come with protective separator sheets between each filter. The color names and the Roscolene filter(s) used to produce that particular color, are printed on a card included with the filters and a set of instructions on how to fit them to a lamp.

Rhino Publishing
www.rhinopublish.com

What Is Going on Here?

Peroxides are supposed to be bad for you. Free radicals and all that. But now we hear that hydrogen peroxide is good for us. Hydrogen peroxide will put extra oxygen in your blood. There's no doubt about that. Hydrogen peroxide costs pennies. So if you can get oxygen into the blood cheaply and safely, maybe cancer (which doesn't like oxygen), emphysema, AIDS, and many other terrible diseases can be treated effectively. Intravenous hydrogen peroxide rapidly relieves allergic reactions, influenza symptoms, and acute viral infections.

No one expects to live forever. But we would all like to have a George Burns finish. The prospect of finishing life in a nursing home after abandoning your tricycle in the mobile home park is not appealing. Then comes the loss of control of vital functions the ultimate humiliation. Is life supposed to be from tricycle to tricycle and diaper to diaper? You come into this world crying, but do you have to leave crying? I don't believe you do. And you won't either after you see the evidence. Sounds too good to be true, doesn't it? Read on and decide for yourself.

-William Campbell Douglass II, MD

Rhino Publishing S.A.
www.rhinopublish.com

HYDROGEN PEROXIDE

Medical Miracle

H_2O

Don't drink your milk!

If you knew what we know about milk... BLEECHT! All that pasteurization, homogenization and processing is not only cooking all the nutrients right out of your favorite drink. It's also adding toxic levels of vitamin D.

This fascinating book tells the whole story about milk. How it once was nature's perfect food...how "raw," unprocessed milk can heal and boost your immune system ... why you can't buy it legally in this country anymore, and what we could do to change that.

Dr. "Douglass traveled all over the world, tasting all kinds of milk from all kinds of cows, poring over dusty research books in ancient libraries far from home, to write this light-hearted but scientifically sound book.

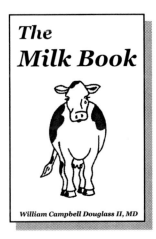

Rhino Publishing, S.A.
www.rhinopublish.com

The
Milk Book

William Campbell Douglass II, MD

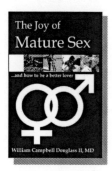

The Joy of Mature Sex
and How to Be a Better Lover

Humans are very confused about what makes good sex. But I believe humans have more to offer each other than this total licentiousness common among animals. We're talking about mature sex. The kind of sex that made this country great.

Stop Aging or Slow the Process
How Exercise With Oxygen Therapy
(EWOT) Can Help

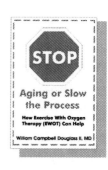

EWOT (pronounced ee-watt) stands for Exercise With Oxygen Therapy. This method of prolonging your life is so simple and you can do it at home at a minimal cost. When your cells don't get enough oxygen, they degenerate and die and so you degenerate and die. It's as simple as that.

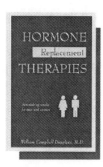

Hormone Replacement Therapies:
Astonishing Results For Men And Women

It is accurate to say that when the endocrine glands start to fail, you start to die. We are facing a sea change in longevity and health in the elderly. Now, with the proper supplemental hormones, we can slow the aging process and, in many cases, reverse some of the signs and symptoms of aging.

Add 10 Years to Your Life
With some "best of" Dr. Douglass' writings.

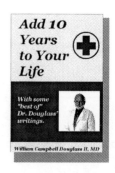

To add ten years to your life, you need to have the right attitude about health and an understanding of the health industry and what it's feeding you. Following the established line on many health issues could make you very sick or worse! Achieve dynamic health with this collection of some of the "best of" Dr. Douglass' newsletters.

How did AIDS become one of the Greatest Biological Disasters in the History of Mankind?

GET THE FACTS

AIDS and BIOLOGICAL WARFARE covers the history of plagues from the past to today's global confrontation with AIDS, the Prince of Plagues. Completely documented *AIDS and BIOLOGICAL WARFARE* helps you make your own decisions about how to survive in a world ravaged by this horrible plague.

You will learn that AIDS is not a naturally occuring disease process as you have been led to believe, but a man-made biological nightmare that has been unleashed and is now threatening the very existence of human life on the planet.

There is a smokescreen of misinformation clouding the AIDS issue. Now, for the first time, learn the truth about the nature of the crisis our planet faces: its origin -- how AIDS is really transmited and alternatives for treatment. Find out what they are not telling you about AIDS and Biological Warfare, and how to protect yourself and your loved ones. AIDS is a serious problem worldwide, but it is no longer the major threat. You need to know the whole story. To protect yourself, you must know the truth about biological warfare.

PAINFUL DILEMMA

Are we fighting the wrong war?

We are spending millions on the war against drugs while we
should be fighting the war against pain with those drugs!

As you will read in this book, the war on drugs was lost a long time ago and,
when it comes to the war against pain, pain is winning! An article in USA Today
(11/20/02) reveals that dying patients are not getting relief from pain. It seems
the doctors are torn between fear of the government, certainly justified, and a
clinging to old and out dated ideas about pain, which is NOT justified.

A group called Last Acts, a coalition of health-care groups, has released a very
discouraging study of all 50 states that nearly half of the 1.6 million Americans
living in nursing homes suffer from untreated pain. They said that life was being
extended but it amounted to little more than "extended pain and suffering."

This book offers insight into the history of pain treatment and the current failed
philosophies of contemporary medicine. Plus it describes some of today's most
advanced treatments for alleviating certain kinds of pain. This book is not another
"self-help" book touting home remedies; rather, Painful Dilemma: Patients in
Pain -- People in Prison, takes a hard look at where we've gone wrong and what
we (you) can do to help a loved one who is living with chronic pain.

The second half of this book is a must read if you value your freedom. We now
have the ridiculous and tragic situation of people
in pain living in a government-created hell by
restriction of narcotics and people in prison for
trying to bring pain relief by the selling of
narcotics to the suffering. The end result of the
"war on drugs" has been to create the greatest
and most destructive cartel in history, so great,
in fact, that the drug Mafia now controls most
of the world economy.

PAINFUL DILEMMA
PATIENTS IN PAIN
PEOPLE IN PRISON

Rhino Publishing S.A.
www.rhinopublish.com

Live the Adventure!

Why would anyone in their right mind put everything they own in storage and move to Russia, of all places?! But when maverick physician Bill Douglass left a profitable medical practice in a peaceful mountaintop town to pursue "pure medical truth".... none of us who know him well was really surprised.

After All, anyone who's braved the outermost reaches of darkest Africa, the mean streets of Johannesburg and New York, and even a trip to Washington to testify before the Senate, wouldn't bat and eye at ducking behind the Iron Curtain for a little medical reconnaissance!

Enjoy this imaginative, funny, dedicated man's tales of wonder and woe as he treks through a year in St. Petersburg, working on a cure for the world's killer diseases. We promise --

YOU WON'T BE BORED!

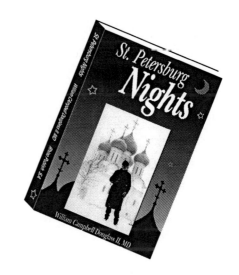

Rhino Publishing S.A.
www.rhinopublish.com

THE SMOKER'S PARADOX
THE HEALTH BENEFITS OF TOBACCO!

The benefits of smoking tobacco have been common knowledge for centuries. From sharpening mental acuity to maintaining optimal weight, the relatively small risks of smoking have always been outweighed by the substantial improvement to mental and physical health. Hysterical attacks on tobacco notwithstanding, smokers always weigh the good against the bad and puff away or quit according to their personal preferences. Now the same anti-tobacco enterprise that has spent billions demonizing the pleasure of smoking is providing additional reasons to smoke. Alzheimer's, Parkinson's, Tourette's Syndrome, even schizophrenia and cocaine addiction are disorders that are alleviated by tobacco. Add in the still inconclusive indication that tobacco helps to prevent colon and prostate cancer and the endorsement for smoking tobacco by the medical establishment is good news for smokers and non-smokers alike. Of course the revelation that tobacco is good for you is ruined by the pharmaceutical industry's plan to substitute the natural and relatively inexpensive tobacco plant with their overpriced and ineffective nicotine substitutions. Still, when all is said and done, the positive revelations regarding tobacco are very good reasons indeed to keep lighting those cigars - but only 4 a day!

THE SMOKER'S PARADOX
William Campbell Douglass II, MD

The health benefits of tobacco

Rhino Publishing, S.A
www.rhinopublish.com

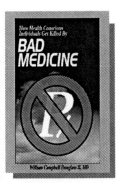

Bad Medicine
How Individuals Get Killed By Bad Medicine.

Do you really need that new prescription or that overnight stay in the hospital? In this report, Dr. Douglass reveals the common medical practices and misconceptions endangering your health. Best of all, he tells you the pointed (but very revealing!) questions your doctor prays you never ask. Interesting medical facts about popular remedies are revealed.

Dangerous Legal Drugs
The Poisons in Your Medicine Chest.

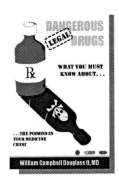

If you knew what we know about the most popular prescription and over-the-counter drugs, you'd be sick. That's why Dr. Douglass wrote this shocking report about the poisons in your medicine chest. He gives you the low-down on different categories of drugs. Everything from painkillers and cold remedies to tranquilizers and powerful cancer drugs.

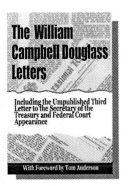

The William Campbell Douglass Letters.
Expose of Government Machinations
(Vietnam War).

THE WILLIAM CAMPBELL DOUGLASS LETTERS. Dr. Douglass' Defense in 1968 Tax Case and Expose of Government Machinations during the Vietnam War.

The Eagle's Feather. A Novel of
International Political Intrigue.

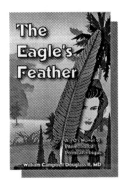

Although The Eagle's Feather is a work of fiction set in the 1970's, it is built, as with most fiction, on a framework of plausibility and background information. This is a fiction book that could not have been written were it not for various ominous aspects, which pose a clear and present danger to the security of the United States.

Rhino Publishing

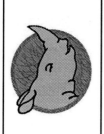

ORDER FORM

PURCHASER INFORMATION

Purchaser's Name (Please Print): _____

Shipping Address (Do not use a P.O. Box): _____

City: _____ State/Prov.: _____ Country: _____

Zip/Postal Code: _____ Telephone No.: _____ Fax No.: _____

E-Mail Address (if interested in receiving free e-Books when available): _____

CREDIT CARD INFO (CIRCLE ONE):

MASTERCARD, VISA, AMERICAN EXPRESS, DISCOVER, JCB, DINER'S CLUB, CARTE BLANCHE.

Charge my Card -> Number #: _____ Exp.: _____

*Security Code: _____ * Required for all MasterCard, Visa and American Express purchases. For your security, we require that you enter your card's verification number. The verification number is also called a CCV number. This code is the 3 digits farthest right in the signature field on the back of your VISA/MC, or the 4 digits to the right on the front of your American Express card. Your credit card statement will show a **different name than Rhino Publishing** as the vendor.

WE DO NOT share your private information, we use 3ʳᵈ party credit card processing service to process your order only.

ADDITIONAL INFORMATION

If your shipping address is not the same as your credit card billing address, please indicate your card billing address here.

_____   _____

Name on the card   Type of card:

Billing Address: _____

City: _____ State/Prov.: _____ Zip/Postal Code: _____

Fax a copy of this order to:
RHINO PUBLISHING, S.A.

1-888-317-6767 or International #: + 416-352-5126

To order by mail, send your payment by first class mail only to the following address. Please include a copy of this order form. Make your check or bank drafts (NO postal money order) payable to RHINO PUBLISHING, S.A. and mail to:

Rhino Publishing, S.A.
Attention: PTY 5048
P.O. Box 025724
Miami, FL.
USA 33102

Digital E-books also available online: www.rhinopublish.com

Rhino
Publishing

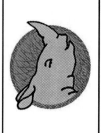

ORDER
FORM

Purchaser's Name (Please Print):

I would like to order the following paperback book of Dr. Douglass (Alternative Medicine Books):

___ X	9962-636-04-3	Add 10 Years to Your Life. With some "best of" Dr. Douglass writings.	$13.99 $ ___
___ X	9962-636-07-8	AIDS and Biological Warfare. What They Are Not Telling You!	$17.99 $ ___
___ X	9962-636-09-4	Bad Medicine. How Individuals Get Killed By Bad Medicine.	$11.99 $ ___
___ X	9962-636-10-8	Color Me Healthy. The Healing Power of Colors.	$11.99 $ ___
___ X	9962-636 -XX-X	Color Filters for Color Me Healthy. 11 Basic Roscolene Filters for Lamps.	$21.89 $ ___
___ X	9962-636-15-9	Dangerous Legal Drugs. The Poisons in Your Medicine Chest.	$13.99 $ ___
___ X	9962-636-18-3	Dr. Douglass' Complete Guide to Better Vision. Improve eyesight naturally.	$11.99 $ ___
___ X	9962-636-19-1	Eat Your Cholesterol! How to Live off the Fat of the Land and Feel Great.	$11.99 $ ___
___ X	9962-636-12-4	Grandma Bell's A To Z Guide To Healing. Her Kitchen Cabinet Cures.	$14.99 $ ___
___ X	9962-636-22-1	Hormone Replacement Therapies. Astonishing Results For Men & Women	$11.99 $ ___
___ X	9962-636-25-6	Hydrogen Peroxide: One of the Most Underused Medical Miracle.	$15.99 $ ___
___ X	9962-636-27-2	Into the Light. New Edition with Blood Irradiation Instrument Instructions.	$19.99 $ ___
___ X	9962-636-54-X	Milk Book. The Classic on the Nutrition of Milk and How to Benefit from it.	$17.99 $ ___

___ X	9962-636-00-0	Painful Dilemma - Patients in Pain - People in Prison.	$17.99 $ ___
___ X	9962-636-32-9	Prostate Problems. Safe, Simple, Effective Relief for Men over 50.	$11.99 $ ___
___ X	9962-636-34-5	St. Petersburg Nights. Enlightening Story of Life and Science in Russia.	$17.99 $ ___
___ X	9962-636-37-X	Stop Aging or Slow the Process. Exercise With Oxygen Therapy Can Help.	$11.99 $ ___
___ X	9962-636-60-4	The Hypertension Report. Say Good Bye to High Blood Pressure.	$11.99 $ ___
___ X	9962-636-48-5	The Joy of Mature Sex and How to Be a Better Lover...	$13.99 $ ___
___ X	9962-636-43-4	The Smoker's Paradox: Health Benefits of Tobacco.	$14.99 $ ___

Political Books:

___ X	9962-636-40-X	The Eagle's Feather. A 70's Novel of International Political Intrigue.	$15.99 $ ___
___ X	9962-636-46-9	The W. C. D. Letters. Expose of Government Machinations (Vietnam War).	$11.99 $ ___
		SUB-TOTAL:	$ ___

ADD $5.00 HANDLING FOR YOUR ORDER: $ 5.00 $ 5.00

___ X ADD $2.50 SHIPPING FOR EACH ITEM ON ORDER: $ 2.50 $ ___

NOTE THAT THE MINIMUM SHIPPING AND HANDLING IS $7.50 FOR 1 BOOK ($5.00 + $2.50)

For order shipped outside the US, add $5.00 per item

___ X ADD $5.00 S. & H. OR EACH ITEM ON ORDER (INTERNATIONAL ORDERS ONLY) $ 5.00 $ ___

Allow up to 21 days for delivery (we will call you about back orders if any)

         TOTAL: $ ___

Fax a copy of this order to: 1-888-317-6767 or Int'l + 416-352-5126
or mail to: Rhino Publishing, S.A. Attention: PTY 5048 P.O. Box 025724, Miami, FL., 33102 USA
Digital E-books also available online: www.rhinopublish.com

CPSIA information can be obtained at www.ICGtesting.com
230302LV00002B/106/A